Ketogenic Fat Bombs
Sweets & Snacks

Volume 2

By Anas Malla

Copyright 2017 - All rights reserved.

This document is geared towards providing exact and reliable information in regards to the topic and issue covered. The publication is sold on the idea that the publisher is not required to render an accounting, officially permitted, or otherwise, qualified services. If advice is necessary, legal or professional, a practiced individual in the profession should be ordered.

- From a Declaration of Principles which was accepted and approved equally by a Committee of the American Bar Association and a Committee of Publishers and Associations.

In no way is it legal to reproduce, duplicate, or transmit any part of this document by either electronic means or in printed format. Recording of this publication is strictly prohibited and any storage of this document is not allowed unless with written permission from the publisher. All rights reserved.

The information provided herein is stated to be truthful and consistent, in that any liability, in terms of inattention or otherwise, by any usage or abuse of any policies, processes, or directions contained within is the solitary and utter responsibility of the recipient reader. Under no circumstances will any legal responsibility or blame be held against the publisher for any reparation, damages, or monetary loss due to the information herein, either directly or indirectly.

Respective authors own all copyrights not held by the publisher.

The information herein is offered for informational purposes solely and is universal as so. The presentation of the information is without a contract or any type of guarantee assurance.

The trademarks that are used are without any consent, and the publication of the trademark is without permission or backing by the trademark owner. All trademarks and brands within this book are for clarifying purposes only and are the owned by the owners themselves, not affiliated with this document.

Bonus!! FREE E-Book

This great book has a Bonus E-book called "10.5 Tips for Massive Success". You can download the book from my website.

I am honored and grateful to give you this free e-book, and I hope this will really help you to start your ketogenic diet, you can easy read it after downloading.

Thank you and enjoy reading.

If the links do not work, for whatever reason, you can simply visit my website:

Mastering-life.com/10successtipsbook

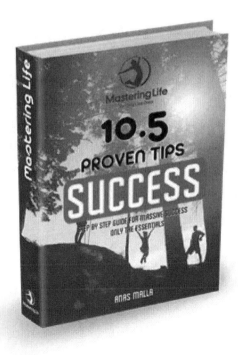

Table of Contents

INTRODUCTION 1

KETOGENIC FAT BOMBS 3
- Keto Mediterranean Fat Bomb 3
- Cinnamon Bars 5
- Coconut Fat Bombs 6
- Ginger Fat Bombs 8
- Lemon Fat Bombs 9
- Buttery Fat Bombs 10
- Blueberry Fat Bombs 12
- Chocolate Fat Bombs 14
- Butter Pecan Fat Bombs with White Chocolate 15
- Simple Orange Butter Fat Bombs 16
- Seasonal Four Spice Fat Bombs 17
- Pumpkin Fat Bombs 18
- Zucchini Bread with Walnuts 19
- Savory Italian Egg Bake 21
- Cheesy Cauliflower Onion Dip 23

KETOGENIC SWEETS RECIPES 27
- Keto Cake Roll 27
- Meringue Custard 30
- Mocha Cheesecake Bars 32
- Choco Silk Pie 34
- Choco Tarts with Peanut Butter 37
- Keto Brownie Fudge 39
- Ketogenic Bounty Bars 41
- Keto Ferrero Rocher 43

Keto Ice Cream 46
 Mint Chip Pudding 48
 Simple Coco-Blueberry Cream 49
 Simple Almond Fudge 50
 Berry Vanilla Jello 51
 Keto Caramel Clusters 52
 Ketogenic Creamsicles 54

KETOGENIC SNACKS RECIPES 57
 Keto Ginger Cookies 57
 Keto Cloud Cakes 59
 Coco-Cashew Bars 61
 Choco Macaroons 62
 Pumpkin Cookies 64
 Blueberry Cookies 65
 Choco Biscuits 67
 Ginger Cookies 69
 Spicy Cookies 71
 Skillet Brownies 73
 Keto Coco Bark 75
 Choco Low-Carb Bar 77
 Cheese Crackers 79
 Ketogenic Nachos 81
 Zucchini Mini Pizza 83

CONCLUSION 84

Introduction

I want to thank you and congratulate you for purchasing the book "**Ketogenic Fat Bombs, Sweets, & Snacks Volume 2**"!

This book contains recipes for fat bombs, sweets, and snacks that perfectly fit your ketogenic diet plan.

If you didn't know, the ketogenic diet is one of the quickest and safest way to get your weight in order. It was never that easy to lose all those extra pounds like with the ketogenic diet.

However, some of the people have problems with finding enough different recipes for their nutrition plan. They say that it is especially tricky with fat bombs. Well, not anymore!

This book offers you exactly 45 recipes and covers:

- **Ketogenic fat bombs** – sweet and salty recipes perfect for everyone
- **Ketogenic sweets** – dessert recipes ideal for indulging your sweet tooth
- **Ketogenic snacks** – if you are looking for a boost of energy of you don't feel quite full after a meal

And much more!

As someone who is on the ketogenic diet, I tried to select the most tasteful recipes that are at the same time easy to prepare. If you are looking for simple fat bombs, sweets and snacks recipes for keto diet, then you can find all that here.

Thanks again for purchasing this book, I hope you enjoy it!

Ketogenic Fat Bombs

Keto Mediterranean Fat Bomb
Serves 5

Ingredients

½ cup full-fat cream cheese

¼ cup butter at room temperature (use ghee alternatively)

4 pitted olives

3 tablespoons chopped herbs (basil, oregano and/or thyme)

4 pieces of drained sun-dried tomatoes

2 crushed garlic cloves

5 tablespoons grated parmesan cheese

Freshly ground black pepper

Salt to taste

Directions

1. Use a knife to cut the butter into little pieces and mix it in a bowl with cream cheese. If it is thick, you can leave it on the counter for about half an hour to soften. Once it softened enough, use a fork to mash it and make sure it is well combined.
2. Add olives and tomatoes. Next, add the herbs and garlic and season it to taste with pepper and salt. Combine the ingredients well.
3. Place it into the refrigerator to cool down for about half an hour.
4. Once the mixture is solid, take it out of the fridge and start making balls. You can use a scooper or a spoon. There should be enough of the mixture to make 5 balls.
5. Roll each ball in Parmesan cheese and set it on a plate. You can serve immediately or keep in the fridge for up to 7 days.

Cinnamon Bars

Serves 2 bars

Ingredients

2/3 teaspoon cinnamon

½ cup creamed coconut

1 tablespoon almond butter

2 tablespoons coconut oil, extra virgin

Directions

1. Use muffin liners or something similar to line a mini loaf pan or a dish.
2. Combine 1/8 teaspoon of cinnamon and creamed coconut in a bowl.
3. Transfer into the liners. The amount is enough for 2 sections of the mini loaf pan.
4. Use another bowl to combine almond butter and 1 tablespoon of coconut oil. Spread it over the coconut mixture and place the pan into the freezer for about 10 minutes.
5. In the meantime, mix 1 tablespoon of coconut oil and ½ teaspoon of cinnamon in another bowl. Sprinkle over the bars and serve. Alternatively, you can leave it in the freezer to further cool down.

Coconut Fat Bombs
Serves 12

Ingredients

1 ½ cup flaked or shredded coconut, unsweetened

¼ cup butter

¼ cup coconut oil, extra virgin

¼ teaspoon vanilla bean powder or cinnamon

Salt to taste

Directions

1. Turn your oven to 350F. Line a baking sheet with parchment paper.
2. Spread the coconut on the sheet and toast in in the oven for about 5 minutes. You should go for a light golden color. Make sure to stir a couple of times to avoid burning.
3. Move the coconut into a blender and make it smooth.
4. Add coconut oil and butter which you should cut into pieces.
5. Add vanilla or cinnamon and salt to your taste. If you are feeling like having something sweet, you can also add a healthy sweetener, such as Stevia or Erythritol.
6. Use molds to make a form of mini muffins from the mixture. You can use a spoon, and you will get around 12 servings as long as you use 1 ½ tablespoons for each fat bomb.
7. Keep it in the fridge for about 30-40 minutes. Once it solidifies, serve the dish.

Ginger Fat Bombs
Serves 10

Ingredients

2.6 oz. softened coconut butter

2.6 oz. coconut oil

1 teaspoon ginger powder

1 oz. shredded coconut

1 teaspoon healthy sweetener (Stevia or Erythritol)

Directions

1. Combine all the ingredients in a bowl. Whisk them well until there are no traces of the sweetener you used.
2. Use a spoon to transfer the mixture into muffin molds and make fat bombs.
3. Put them in the fridge for 15-20 minutes before serving.

Lemon Fat Bombs
Serves 16

Ingredients

7 oz. softened coconut butter

¼ cup coconut oil, extra virgin

Fresh lemon zest from 1 or 2 lemons

Salt to taste

15-20 drops of Erythritol or another healthy sweetener per your choice

Directions

1. Soften the coconut butter and the coconut oil to room temperature. Use a grater to make the lemon zest. You don't want large pieces of the zest in your fat bombs.
2. Combine all the ingredients in one bowl. You should evenly distribute the lemon zest and sweetener. The amount of sweetener to use is just a suggestion, make it sweet or salty per your taste.
3. Use a spoon to transfer the mixture into molds or mini muffin paper cups.
4. Put in in the fridge for about 60 minutes to solidify. You can keep it in the fridge for up to 7 days, but make sure not to keep it at room temperature for long because the coconut oil and butter will get soft.

Buttery Fat Bombs
Serves 8

Ingredients

8 oz. almond butter, unsweetened

8 oz. coconut butter, raw

1 stick and 2 tablespoons of butter

1 bar 90% cocoa dark chocolate

Erythritol or another sweetener of your choice

Directions

1. Place coconut butter, almond butter and the stick of the regular butter into a microwave-safe bowl. Melt it for 30 seconds at a time until they are soft enough to be easily mixed.
2. Add the sweetener and make sure to stir it well. You can also add roasted nuts or unsweetened dried fruits.
3. Pour the mixture into silicone molds or muffin cups and place them into the fridge to cool down for about 30-45 minutes.
4. In the meantime, melt the chocolate in the microwave along with the remaining 2 tablespoons of butter.
5. When your butter mixture is cool and solid, take it out of the fridge and dip it into melted chocolate.
6. Let the fat bombs cool down a bit on a baking sheet and return them to the fridge.
7. Serve cold and make sure not to keep it long at room temperature because the coconut butter will melt.

Blueberry Fat Bombs

Serves 12-24 (depending on the size of the molds you use)

Ingredients

1 cup blueberries

4 oz. butter (1 stick)

¾ cup coconut oil

¼ cup coconut cream

4 oz. softened cream cheese

Optional sweetener

Directions

1. Take out your candy molds and place 3 or 4 blueberries into each of them (depending on the size of the mold you use).
2. Use the saucepan to melt coconut oil and butter over low heat. Allow it to cool down a bit.
3. Add all the other ingredients to the butter mixture and make sure to combine them well. You can even use a blender to make the process easier. If you want, you can add sweetener to your taste.
4. Pour the mixture over the blueberries in the molds. Make sure not to fill them all the way to the top.
5. Place the fat bombs into the fridge for an hour or two before serving.

Alternative Directions for the Pureed Version

1. Put berries, cream cheese and coconut cream into a blender to make the mixture smooth.
2. Use a saucepan to melt the coconut oil and butter over low heat. Allow it to cool down a bit.
3. Put the butter mixture into the blender and puree one more time.
4. If you want, add the sweetener and make sure you stir it in well.
5. Transfer the mixture into silicone candy molds and put it in the fridge for about an hour before serving.

Chocolate Fat Bombs
Serves 14

Ingredients

4.5 oz. coconut oil

1 oz. unsweetened cocoa powder

1 tablespoon tahini paste

1 tablespoon Erythritol or another sweetener of your choice

1 oz. walnut halves

Directions

1. Heat the pan over low-medium heat to melt the coconut oil.
2. Move it into a bowl and add all the remaining ingredients.
3. Allow the mixture to cool down slightly.
4. Transfer the mixture into muffin cups or candy molds. Fill about one-half of each mold.
5. Put a half walnut over each fat bomb to decorate.

Butter Pecan Fat Bombs with White Chocolate

Serves 4

Ingredients

2 oz. cocoa butter

2 tablespoons butter

2 tablespoons coconut oil

½ cup chopped pecans

¼ teaspoon vanilla extract

2 tablespoons Erythritol

A pinch of salt

Directions

1. Use a small pan to melt cocoa butter, coconut oil, and butter over low heat. Allow it to cool down a bit.
2. Add the Erythritol or sweetener of your choice. Follow it with just a pinch of salt to balance the sweetness. Next, stir in the vanilla extract.
3. Add a couple of chopped pecans (I suggest no more than 4) into each of the candy molds or ice cube trays you use.
4. Pour the butter mixture over the pecans.
5. Place it into the freezer for 30-45 minutes to serve cold.

Simple Orange Butter Fat Bombs
Serves 2

Ingredients

1 oz. cream cheese

4 pecan halves

½ teaspoon of finely grated orange zest

½ tablespoon unsalted butter

Salt to taste

Directions

1. Turn your oven to 350F and toast the pecans for up to 10 minutes. Allow them to cool.
2. In the meantime, soften the cream cheese and the butter. Add orange zest and combine the ingredients well.
3. Spread the orange mixture between pecan halves. If you want, sprinkle with sea salt and serve.

Seasonal Four Spice Fat Bombs
Serves 6

Ingredients

8 oz. cream cheese

1 teaspoon ginger

1 tablespoon cinnamon

½ teaspoon nutmeg

½ teaspoon ground cloves

¾ cups coconut oil

½ cup stevia

Directions

1. Use a food processor to blend all the ingredients except the oil. Make sure to process slowly, while slowly pouring in the coconut oil.
2. Divide the mixture into 6 chunks and make the form of a ball out of each of them.
3. Place it in the fridge for about 15 minutes.
4. You can put melted dark chocolate (sugar-free) over the balls to get a better taste. In this case, return to the refrigerator to further cool down.

Pumpkin Fat Bombs

Serves 20 (depending on the size of the balls)

Ingredients

½ cup pumpkin

4 tablespoons unsalted butter

2 tablespoons coconut oil

Clove

Ginger

Nutmeg

Cinnamon

Stevia

Directions

1. Use a small saucepan to melt the coconut oil over medium heat.
2. Add butter and combine the ingredients well.
3. Slowly stir in the pumpkins. Combine until you get a creamy and smooth mixture. Add stevia and spices.
4. Line a baking sheet with parchment paper. Transfer the mixture to the sheet. Put it in the fridge to solidify (for about 15 minutes).
5. Take it out of the fridge and make balls out of the mixture. If you make around 1" size balls, you should have about 20 balls.
6. Keep it in the fridge for about one hour to solidify before serving.

Zucchini Bread with Walnuts
Serves 16

Ingredients

1/4 teaspoon. of ground ginger

1/2 teaspoon. of salt

1/2 cup of olive oil

1/2 teaspoon. of nutmeg

1/2 cup of chopped walnuts

1 teaspoon. of ground cinnamon

1 teaspoon. of vanilla extract

1 cup of grated zucchini

1 1/2 cup of Erythritol

1 1/2 teaspoon. of baking powder

2 1/2 cup of almond flour

3 eggs

Directions

1. Preheat your oven to 350°F. mix oil, vanilla extract, and eggs. Then set that to the side.
2. Take another bowl and mix almond flour, salt, Erythritol, nutmeg, baking powder, ginger, and cinnamon. Also set to the side.
3. Using a paper towel or cheesecloth, take the zucchini and squeeze out the excess water.
4. Mix the zucchini into the bowl with eggs.
5. Then, add the dry ingredients slowly into the mixture with eggs. Use a hand mixer until it's fully blended.
6. Lightly spray a loaf pan (9x5) and spoon in the zucchini mixture.
7. On the top of the zucchini bread spoon in the walnuts. Use a spatula to press walnuts into the batter.
1. 8.Bake it for 60-70 minutes at 350°F (or the walnuts on top look browned).

Savory Italian Egg Bake
Serves 8

Ingredients

1/2 cup of heavy whipping cream

1/2 cup of tomato sauce

1/2 cup grated Parmesan cheese

1 teaspoon. of parsley flakes

1 cup of extra sharp cheese, shredded

2 cup of cooked chicken breast, diced

2 teaspoon. of garlic and her seasonings

3 tablespoons. of mustard

10 large eggs

12 oz. of frozen broccoli florets

Directions

1. Preheat oven to 350°F. Mix the eggs together in a large mixing bowl.
2. Mix in garlic and herb seasoning, the mustard and heavy whipping cream.
3. When it's all blended well slowly add in the tomato sauce until it's no longer lumpy and then add broccoli florets and diced chicken.
4. Grease a large baking pan or a casserole dish and then pour in the Italian bake.
5. Sprinkle parsley flakes and Parmesan cheese on top of the Italian bake. Bake at 350°F for 30-40 minutes (or until the top looks like a crust)
6. Top the Italian bake with some extra sharp cheese before serving (or any other cheese, for example mozzarella, pepper jack ketchup).

Cheesy Cauliflower Onion Dip
Serves 24

Ingredients

3/4 cup of cream cheese

1/4 cup of mayonnaise

1/2 cup of medium sized onion

1/2 teaspoon. of salt

1/2 teaspoon. of ground, black pepper

1/2 teaspoon. of garlic powder

1/2 teaspoon. of chili powder

1/2 teaspoon. of ground cumin

1 pound of cauliflower

1 1/2 cup of chicken broth

Directions

1. Simmer half and onion and the cauliflower in chicken broth until it's soft and tender. Stir in chili powder, cumin, pepper and salt and garlic powder.
2. Mix chunks of cream cheese (after cutting them up) into the cauliflower until the cream cheese melts, and it's no longer chunky.
3. Use a regular blender, or a stick blender if you have one, to blend the mixture until it's smooth.
4. Carefully mix in the mayonnaise. Before serving chill in the fridge for 2-3 hours.

Get FREE Access To "11 Ketogenic Food Lists"

Go to: http://bit.ly/2pa7IrX

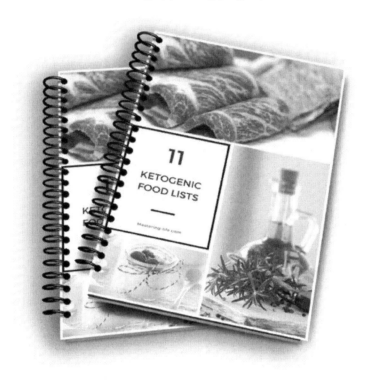

Ketogenic Sweets Recipes

Keto Cake Roll
Serves 10

Ingredients

3 big eggs

1 cup almond flour

½ cup heavy whipping cream

¼ cup matcha powder

¼ cup psyllium husk powder

1 teaspoon baking powder

½ cup Swerve or sweetener of your choice

1 teaspoon vanilla

4 tablespoons melted butter

Salt to taste

Filling:

¼ cup Swerve or sweetener of your choice

1 pack gelatin, unflavored

2 cups heavy whipping cream

2 teaspoon vanilla

Directions

1. Turn your oven to 350F to preheat it. Grab a big bowl and add matcha powder, psyllium husk powder, almond flour, baking powder, Swerve or sweetener of your choice, and salt to it. Combine all the ingredients well. You don't want to have any lumps in your batter.
2. Use a different bowl to add eggs, butter, vanilla, and heavy whipping cream. Combine all the ingredients well and once they are mixed, add them to the flour mixture. Once again, combine everything well until you get a thick dough.
3. Use parchment paper to line up a baking sheet. Arrange the dough on it in the form of a big rectangle. The dough should be pretty flat. Bake for 10 minutes at the set temperature. Allow it to cool down a bit.
4. Once it's cool enough to handle you can use parchment paper to roll the dough up. You will need to be very gentle. Don't make it extra tight.

5. While the dough is cooling down, make the filling by grabbing a bowl and adding 4 tablespoons of lukewarm water to it. Next, add a pack of gelatin and allow it to sit for about 4-5 minutes. Put it in the microwave for 15 seconds to warm it up and stir the ingredients well. Add heavy whipping cream and vanilla and use an electric hand mixer to combine until you get a thick filling.
6. Unroll the cake carefully and spread the mixture over it. Once again, use parchment paper to roll it back up. Place it in the freezer for at least 15 minutes to cool down before serving.

Meringue Custard
Serves 4

Ingredients

2 egg whites

1 tablespoon Swerve or sweetener of your choice

1/8 teaspoon tartar cream

1/8 teaspoon vanilla extract

Custard:

2 egg yolks

1/3 cup Swerve or sweetener of your choice

½ teaspoon lemon extract

½ teaspoon vanilla extract

1 ½ cups heavy whipping cream

½ teaspoon xanthan gum

2 lemons' zest

Salt to taste

Directions

1. Use a saucepan and add xanthan gum, lemon zest, Swerve or sweetener of your choice, and salt to it. Combine everything together and add a tablespoon of heavy whipping cream.

2. Place on the stove and whisk everything together. Heat the mixture over low temperature and slowly add the remaining heavy whipping cream. Make sure to mix everything constantly.
3. Next, add egg yolks and increase the temperature to medium, allowing the mixture to start to simmer, but making sure that you continue stirring. Once you see that it's simmering, remove from the stove and put on the counter.
4. Add lemon and vanilla extract and stir everything together once again. Use ramekins and arrange the mixture evenly across them (you will need four).
5. Use a bowl to combine egg whites and tartar cream with an electric hand mixer. You want the mixture to form a soft peak. Add Swerve or sweetener of your choice and vanilla. Continue mixing with the mixer until it forms a stiff peak.
6. Divide the meringue mixture evenly across the ramekins and over the custard. You can use your spoon to press down a bit and then lift it upward briskly to make a peak.
7. Bake for about 30 seconds in your broiler set to high temperature. Your goal is to get the peaks of meringue brown, but avoid over-browning it. Allow it to cool down before serving.

Mocha Cheesecake Bars
Serves 16

Ingredients

3 big eggs

6 tablespoons butter

1 cup Swerve or sweetener of your choice

2 cups almond flour

½ cup cocoa for baking

½ tablespoon instant coffee

1 tsp. baking powder

2 teaspoons vanilla extract

½ teaspoon salt

Cheesy Layer:

½ cup Swerve or sweetener of your choice

1 lb. cream cheese

1 big egg

1 tsp. vanilla extract

Directions

1. Turn your oven to 350F to preheat it and use parchment paper to line a baking pan and cooking spray to grease it.
2. Grab a bowl and add vanilla extract and butter. Combine it well and then add the eggs. Continue mixing until everything is combined.
3. Use a different and add instant coffee, almond flour, baking cocoa, Swerve or sweetener of your choice, baking powder, and salt to it. Combine everything well.
4. Next, add the egg-butter mixture to the flour mix and combine all the ingredients well. Take out ¼ cup of dough and save it for later. Arrange the dough on the baking pan.
5. Use a bowl to mix egg, cream cheese, Swerve or sweetener of your choice, and vanilla extract. Spread the mixture over the arranged dough on the baking pan. Use the remaining batter to top the cheesy layer and make a top crust.
6. Bake for 30 minutes at the set temperature. Allow it to cool down before serving.

Choco Silk Pie
Serves 10

Ingredients

1 egg

1 ½ cup almond flour

1/3 cup Swerve or sweetener of your choice

1 ½ teaspoon vanilla extract

½ teaspoon baking powder

3 tablespoons butter

1/8 teaspoon salt

Filling:

1 cup heavy whipping cream

16 ounces cream cheese

½ cup + 2 teaspoons Swerve or sweetener of your choice

½ cup cocoa powder

4 tablespoons butter

4 tablespoons sour cream

1 tablespoon + 1 teaspoon vanilla extract

Directions

1. Turn your oven to 375F to preheat it. Use cooking spray to grease a baking pan.
2. Grab a bowl and add almond flour, Swerve or sweetener of your choice, salt, and baking powder. Combine the ingredients well.
3. Add butter and use a fork or a pastry blender to mash the mixture and make coarse crumbs. Add vanilla extract and egg and continue mixing until you form a ball from the dough.
4. Arrange the batter on the baking pan evenly. You can use your fingers to cover all the sides of the pan. You should also poke holes in the crust to keep the dough from making bubbles during baking.
5. Bake for 11 minutes at the set temperature. Take the pie out of the oven and use aluminum foil to cover the edges. Bake for additional 7 minutes. Allow it to cool down.
6. In the meantime, make the filling by taking a bowl and adding sour cream, ½ cup of Swerve or sweetener of your choice, cocoa powder, 1 tablespoon vanilla extract, cream cheese, and butter. Use an electric hand mixer to combine all the ingredients well. Your goal is to make a fluffy mixture.

7. Use a different bowl to combine the remaining vanilla extract and Swerve or sweetener of your choice along with the heavy whipping cream. Once combined, gradually add the mixture to the cream cheese mix. You should combine all the ingredients while keeping the bubbles in the cream.
8. Spread the filling over the pie (you can use a spoon or a scoop). Place it in the fridge for 3 hours to cool down. Serve cold.

Choco Tarts with Peanut Butter
Serves 4

Ingredients

2 tablespoons almond flour

1 big egg white

¼ cup + 1 tablespoon Swerve or sweetener of your choice

¼ cup flaxseeds

2 tablespoons butter

4 tablespoons peanut butter

2 tablespoons heavy whipping cream

½ teaspoon cinnamon

4 tablespoons cocoa powder

½ teaspoon vanilla extract

1 avocado

Directions

1. Turn your oven to 350F to preheat it. Use a grinder or a food processor to blend the flax seeds until you get a crumbly mixture.
2. Grab a bowl and add the flax seeds, 1 tablespoon of Swerve or sweetener of your choice, egg white, and almond flour. Arrange the mixture on the tart pans and bake for 8 minutes at the set temperature. Allow it to cool down.
3. In the meantime, use a blender or a food processor and add avocado, cocoa powder, ¼ cup of Swerve or sweetener of your choice, vanilla extract, cinnamon, and heavy whipping cream to it. Process the mix until you get a smooth consistency.
4. Use a heatproof bowl to combine butter with peanut butter. Put it in the microwave for 15 to 20 seconds (more if needed) until the mixture is soft. Once the baked crust cools down, spread the melted mixture over it. Place it in the refrigerator and cool it down for at least 45 minutes.
5. Once the tart is cool, spread the avocado layer over it and cool it down for another 45 minutes before serving.

Keto Brownie Fudge
Serves 36

Ingredients

3 eggs

1 cup almond flour

1 cup maple syrup

2 tablespoons vanilla syrup

2 tablespoons ghee

5 ounces dark chocolate

½ cup coconut oil

1 tablespoon peanut butter

Salt to taste

Directions

1. Turn your oven to 375F to preheat it. Grab a medium pot and boil water in it. Grab a heatproof bowl and place it on top as a double boiler. Add ghee, dark chocolate, peanut butter, and coconut oil to the pan and melt everything together.
2. Once the mixture is melted, transfer the bowl to the counter and gradually add all the other ingredients. Make sure to continue mixing while adding them one at a time.
3. Use parchment paper to line a baking pan. Arrange the dough over the pan. Bake for 25 minutes at the set temperature. Allow it to cool down in the fridge for at least three hours. Cut into squares before serving.

Ketogenic Bounty Bars
Serves 6

Ingredients

8 ounces dark chocolate

½ cup Swerve or sweetener of your choice

1/3 cup coconut milk

1/3 cup coconut oil

1 cup coconut, shredded

Directions

1. Use a saucepan and add coconut milk, Swerve or sweetener of your choice, and coconut oil to it. Turn the temperature on low to melt the coconut oil, but make sure to stir to keep it from burning constantly.
2. Add the coconut and continue mixing until you combine all the ingredients. Use parchment paper to line a loaf pan. Divide the mixture evenly across the bottom of the pan. Put it in the fridge for at least 3 hours to solidify.
3. Remove it from the fridge and turn the pan upside down so that you can pop the solid mixture out. Use a knife to cut it into pieces that look like bars.
4. Next, chop the chocolate and melt 3 ounces of it in a double boiler or a pot filled with water. Make sure to stir the mixture occasionally. Remove from the heat and add one ounce of the remaining chocolate to the mix. Your goal is to get a smooth consistency.
5. Place the bars you melted into the dark chocolate and arrange them on a cooling rack. Melt the remaining dark chocolate the same way as the first half of it (read the previous step).
6. Once again, dip the bars into the melted chocolate and return them to the cooling rack. Once the chocolate sets, you can serve the bars.

Keto Ferrero Rocher
Serves 12

Ingredients

¼ cup hazelnuts, chopped

12 hazelnuts

2 ounces dark chocolate

Homemade Nutella:

¼ cup cocoa powder

2 cups hazelnuts

1 tablespoon coconut oil

¼ cup water

¼ cup heavy cream

½ cup Erythritol

1 teaspoon vanilla extract

¼ teaspoon of salt

Directions

1. We will make homemade Nutella first. Turn your oven to 325F to preheat it. Spread hazelnuts on dry cookie sheet. Make sure to distribute them evenly.
2. Roast the hazelnuts for approximately 12 minutes until their skin becomes almost black. Allow them to cool down a bit.
3. Use a kitchen towel and spread the hazelnuts over one-half of the towel. Fold the other half and rub them to take most of the skin off.
4. Place the hazelnuts into a food processor or a blender. You want to make them look like peanut butter. If you notice that the nuts are sticking to the sides too much, add a tablespoon of mild tasting oil (preferably coconut) and repeat the process.
5. Add the other ingredients and blend for a few more times while scraping the sides in between. The processing is done when you get a mixture that reminds you of the original Nutella. Place it in the fridge for at least 30 minutes
6. Now, let's make Ferrero Rocher. Use a dry skillet and add hazelnuts to it. Toast them until they become fragrant. Allow them to cool down.

7. Use parchment paper to line a baking sheet. Grab a teaspoon of Nutella and place it on the sheet. Use a spoon to flatten it to get a form of a small pancake. Place a hazelnut over it and then put another teaspoon of Nutella over it. Use your hand to form a ball from the mixture. Repeat until no hazelnuts are remaining (you should make 12 cookies). Place it in the fridge for at least 30 minutes.
8. Put the dark chocolate into a saucepan and melt it over low-medium heat. Add chopped hazelnuts and combine all the ingredients well.
9. Once the cookies are cool, dip the in the choco-hazelnut mixture. Arrange them on the baking sheet and place them in the fridge to cool down.

Keto Ice Cream
Serves 8

Ingredients

8 ounces cream cheese

2 cups strawberries

1 cup Swerve or sweetener of your choice

1 teaspoon liquid stevia, strawberry flavor (or any of your choice)

Directions

1. Use a blender of a food processor and add strawberries, lemon juice, ½ cup of Swerve or sweetener of your choice, ½ teaspoon of liquid stevia, vanilla extract, and salt to it. Process everything until you get a smooth consistency. Transfer to a bowl and save for later.
2. Now, add half & half and cream cheese and use an electric hand mixer to combine the ingredients until you get a smooth consistency. Add heavy whipping cream, ½ cup of Swerve or sweetener of your choice, and ½ teaspoon of liquid stevia. Continue mixing until you get a smooth consistency.
3. Use an ice cream machine and pour the half & half mixture into it. Follow the device instructions until you get a serving texture.
4. Add strawberry mix to the ice cream and stir everything. If you want, you can keep some of the strawberry mixture for the topping. Put the ice cream in the freezer for at least 3 hours. Serve cold.

Mint Chip Pudding
Serves 3

Ingredients

1 avocado

1 can coconut milk

10 drops Swerve or sweetener of your choice

1 teaspoon peppermint oil

3 drops Stevia

1 tablespoon cacao powder

½ cup coconut oil

Directions

1. Grab a bowl and add cacao powder, Stevia, and coconut oil to it. Combine everything until you get a smooth consistency. Transfer the mix into a container and put it in the fridge for at least 60 minutes. Use a knife to cut the mixture into chips.
2. In the meantime, use a food processor or a blender and add coconut milk, avocado, Swerve or sweetener of your choice, and peppermint oil to it. Process everything until you get a smooth consistency. Add the cut chips and put them into the mixture. Place it in the freezer for at least 60 minutes and serve cold.

Simple Coco-Blueberry Cream
Serves 2

Ingredients

1 cup dark chocolate chips

1 cup raspberries (or any berries you choose)

1 can coconut milk

Directions

1. Make sure to use cold coconut milk for the recipe. Use a scoop to remove the thick part of it (you can leave the water in the can).
2. Add the milk to a bowl and use an electric hand mixer to process for at least 2 minutes. Gradually add berries and stir the ingredients to combine everything. Top with chocolate chips before serving.

Simple Almond Fudge
Serves 1

Ingredients

¼ cup coconut milk

1 cup almond butter

1 teaspoon vanilla extract

1 cup coconut oil

1 teaspoon Swerve or sweetener of your choice

Directions

1. Use a small saucepan and add coconut oil and almond butter to it. Place it on the stove over low temperature and melt the oil.
2. Remove from the heat and add vanilla extract, coconut milk, and Swerve or sweetener of your choice to it. Combine all the ingredients well. Place it in the fridge for at least 3 hours before serving.

Berry Vanilla Jello
Serves 2

2 packs berry jello (sugar-free, use any flavor you like)

3 tablespoons Swerve or sweetener of your choice

2 tablespoons gelatin powder

1 cup heavy whipping cream

1 teaspoon vanilla extract

Ingredients

1. Use a heatproof bowl and add the two packs of berry jello to it. Add a cup of boiling water and stir until you completely dissolve the jello. Add a cup of cold water and stir everything once again. Put in the fridge for at least 60 minutes to cool down.
2. In the meantime, add Swerve or sweetener of your choice, gelatin powder, and vanilla extract to a heatproof bowl. Add heavy whipping cream and combine everything until you mix the ingredients. Add a cup of boiling water and mix until you dissolve the sweetener. Next, insert the heavy whipping cream.
3. Use a silicon mold and add a half of the vanilla mixture into it. Cut the cold berry jello into cubes and place the over the vanilla mix. Finally, top with the remaining vanilla mix. Put the mold into the refrigerator for at least 2 hours. Serve cold.

Keto Caramel Clusters
Serves 9

Ingredients

20 macadamias

9 pecans

1 ½ ounce dark chocolate

9 caramel candies (sugar-free)

3 tablespoons heavy cream

¼ teaspoon vanilla extract

Salt to taste

Directions

1. Turn your oven to 320F to preheat it. Use parchment paper to line a baking sheet. Place pecans equally across the baking sheet and put a couple of macadamia nuts close to each of them. They can even slightly overlap.
2. Arrange caramel candies across the nuts and bake for 10 minutes at the set temperature. Allow it to cool down to let the candies harden a bit.
3. In the meantime, use a pot to melt heavy cream at low temperature. Add dark chocolate and melt everything but make sure to stir gently to prevent from burning. Your goal is to make a smooth consistency.
4. Distribute about a teaspoon of dark chocolate mixture over the nuts and add a bit of salt over it. Place it in the fridge for at least 60 minutes to cool down.

Ketogenic Creamsicles
Serves 4

Ingredients

2 ounces pistachios

8 ounces strawberries

2 spoons Swerve or sweetener of your choice

½ cup almond milk

½ cup heavy whipping cream

Directions

1. You will need popsicle molds for this recipe. Place them in the freezer to chill. Use a bowl and add almond milk, Swerve or sweetener of your choice, strawberries, and heavy whipping cream to it. Blend everything until the ingredients are thoroughly combined.
2. Add pistachios and use a spoon to stir them into the mixture. If you don't like pistachios or they are expensive, use pecans, cashews, or walnuts.
3. Transfer the mixture into the molds and freeze for at least 3 hours before serving.

Get FREE Access To

"30 Days Ketogenic Plan"

Printable – Table

Go to: http://bit.ly/2pVjqJ7

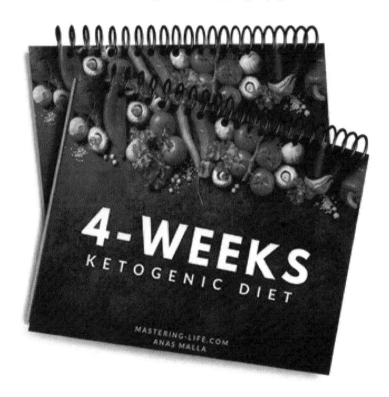

Ketogenic Snacks Recipes

Keto Ginger Cookies
Serves 24

Ingredients

1 cup Swerve or sweetener of your choice

1 big egg

¼ cup butter

2 cups almond flour

1 teaspoon vanilla extract

2 teaspoons ground ginger

½ teaspoon ground cinnamon

¼ teaspoon ground cloves

¼ teaspoon ground nutmeg

Salt to taste

Directions

1. Turn your oven to 350F to preheat it. Use parchment paper to line a baking sheet.
2. Grab a bowl and add egg, butter, and vanilla extract to it. Mix everything until you combine the ingredients well.
3. Use another bowl to combine all the other ingredients (almond flour, Swerve or sweetener of your choice, ground ginger, ground nutmeg, ground cloves, ground cinnamon and salt to taste).
4. Once everything is combined, add the egg mixture to the flour mixture. Use an electric hand mixer to combine all the ingredients well. Don't worry if you get a crisp or stiff batter.
5. Grab a tablespoon of the mixture and place it on the baking sheet. Use the spoon to flatten the cookie. Continue until there is no more batter remaining.
6. Bake for 11 minutes at the set temperature. Allow it to cool down before serving.

Keto Cloud Cakes
Serves 8

Ingredients

6 big eggs

¼ cup Swerve or sweetener of your choice

½ teaspoon tartar cream

6 tablespoons cream cheese

2 teaspoons vanilla extract

Topping:

1/3 cup Swerve or sweetener of your choice

2 tablespoons butter

16 ounces cream cheese

1 tablespoon vanilla extract

Directions

1. Turn your oven to 300F to preheat it. Grease 2 muffin tins with cooking spray.
2. Use two bowls to separate the eggs – place the whites in one of them and the yolks in the other. Add cream cheese, Swerve or sweetener of your choice, and vanilla extract to the bowl with yolks. Use an electric hand mixer to combine everything until you get a smooth consistency.
3. Add tartar cream to the whites and mix until it forms a stiff peak. Slowly add the whites' mixture to the bowl with yolks, but make sure that you don't deflate the whites.
4. Place two tablespoons of the combined mix into each of the tins. Bake for 35 minutes at the set temperature. Allow it to cool down.
5. In the meantime, make the topping by mixing Swerve or sweetener of your choice, cream cheese, butter, and vanilla extract in a bowl. Use an electric hand mixer to combine all the ingredients until you get a smooth consistency.
6. Prepare three layers for each of the cakes. Use a piping bag to add frosting between every layer and form a cake.

Coco-Cashew Bars
Serves 8

Ingredients

½ cup cashews

1 cup almond flour

¼ cup coconut, shredded

¼ cup maple syrup

¼ cup melted butter

1 teaspoon cinnamon

Salt to taste

Directions

1. Grab a big bowl and add almond flour and melted butter to it. Combine the ingredients well.
2. Add maple syrup, cinnamon, shredded coconut, and salt to taste. Combine everything together once again.
3. Chop the cashews and add them to the dough. Once again, mix everything well.
4. Use parchment paper to line a baking sheet. Arrange the batter evenly over the sheet. Put it in the fridge for at least 2 hours to cool down. Cut into bars and serve cold.

Choco Macaroons
Serves 12

Ingredients

1 big egg white

¼ cup dark chocolate chips

½ teaspoon almond extract

1 cup coconut, shredded

¼ cup Swerve or sweetener of your choice

2 tablespoons coconut oil

Salt to taste

Directions

1. Turn your oven to 350F to preheat it. Use parchment paper to line a baking sheet.
2. Spread shredded coconut on the sheet. Bake for 5 minutes at the set temperature to toast the coconut.
3. In the meantime, add the egg white to a bowl and use and electric hand mixer to beat it until it gets foamy. Add Swerve or sweetener of your choice, almond extract, and salt to taste and mix everything well.
4. Next, add the toasted coconut to the mix and fold them in gently. Use a scoop to transfer the balls of the batter on the baking sheet. Bake for 15 minutes at the set temperature.
5. In the meantime, melt dark chocolate and the coconut oil in a small saucepan over medium-low temperature. Make sure to stir frequently to prevent it from burning. Once the cookies are baked, top with the chocolate and serve.

Pumpkin Cookies
Serves 24

Ingredients

2 big eggs

1 ¼ cup pumpkin puree

1 cup almond flour

2 teaspoon garam masala

2 teaspoon cinnamon

1 teaspoon baking powder

1 teaspoon vanilla extract

¼ cup pumpkin pie spice

¼ cup butter

Directions

1. Turn your oven to 350F to preheat it. Use parchment paper to line a baking sheet.
2. Add pumpkin puree, almond flour, baking powder, vanilla extract, butter, and pumpkin pie spice to a food processor or a blender. Process everything until you mix the ingredients well.
3. Spread the mixture evenly on the baking sheet. Use garam masala and cinnamon to adjust it to taste. Bake for 25 minutes at the set temperature.

Blueberry Cookies
Serves 20

Ingredients

½ cup flaxseed meal

8 ounces cream cheese

3 cups almond meal

2 big eggs

8 tablespoons butter

2 tablespoons blueberries

2 cups Swerve or sweetener of your choice

½ teaspoon baking powder

1 vanilla bean seeds

Salt to taste

Directions

1. Turn your oven to 350F to preheat it. Use parchment paper to line a baking pan.
2. Grab a bowl and add almond meal, flaxseed meal, baking powder, vanilla bean seeds, Swerve or sweetener of your choice, cream cheese, butter, eggs, and salt to taste. Combine all the ingredients well.
3. Transfer the batter to the baking pan with a spatula. Make sure to spread it evenly. Use blueberries and spread them over the dough. Bake for 30 minutes at the set temperature. Allow them to cool down before serving.

Choco Biscuits
Serves 15

Ingredients

1 ¾ cups almond flour

1/3 cup Swerve or sweetener of your choice

1 big egg

¼ cup butter

½ cup cocoa, unsweetened

1 teaspoon cinnamon

½ teaspoon vanilla extract

¼ teaspoon xanthan gum

1/3 teaspoon stevia powder

½ teaspoon vanilla extract

Salt to taste

Directions

1. Turn your oven to 325F to preheat it. Use cooking spray to grease a baking sheet or a pan.
2. Grab a bowl and add Swerve or sweetener of your choice, butter, stevia powder, vanilla extract, and egg. Mix until you combine the ingredients well.
3. Use a different bowl and add xanthan gum, almond flour, unsweetened cocoa, cinnamon, and salt to taste. Combine everything well.
4. Combine the ingredients from two bowls and blend them well together. Optionally, you can add nuts or chocolate chips to the mixture.
5. Make a big ball from the dough and place it on the baking sheet. Use your hands to form a log from the batter.
6. Bake for 20 minutes at the set temperature. Reduce the heat to 275F and bake for another 10 minutes. Remove from the oven, allow the dough to cool down a bit and cut it into pieces that remind of biscuits. Bake for additional 25 minutes at the set temperature.

Ginger Cookies
Serves 15

Ingredients

1 egg

½ cup Swerve or sweetener of your choice

1 cup coconut butter

1 teaspoon turmeric powder

1 teaspoon vanilla extract

¼ teaspoon baking soda

2 teaspoons ground ginger

Salt and pepper to taste

Directions

1. Use a food processor or a blender and add vanilla extract, egg, and coconut butter to it. Blend the ingredients until you combine them well.
2. Add ginger, turmeric powder, baking soda, Swerve or sweetener of your choice, and salt and pepper to taste. Blend once again until you combine all the ingredients.
3. Use parchment paper to line a baking sheet. Use your hands to form balls from the dough and arrange them on the sheet. Make a cookie like form by pressing each ball with a spatula or your palm.
4. Bake for 15 minutes at 350F. Allow them to cool down and harden a bit before serving.

Spicy Cookies
Serves 15

Ingredients

1 egg

2 tablespoons chia seeds

2 cups almonds

6 tablespoons Swerve or sweetener of your choice

2 tablespoons cinnamon powder

3 tablespoons ginger, grated

¼ cup coconut oil

½ teaspoon nutmeg

Salt to taste

Directions

1. Turn your oven to 350F to preheat it. Use a blender or a food processor and add chia seeds and almonds to it. Process the ingredients until you blend them together.
2. Use a big bowl and add Swerve or sweetener of your choice, cinnamon powder, ginger, nutmeg, coconut oil, chia-almond mixture, and salt to taste to it. Use an electric hand mixer to combine all the ingredients together.
3. Use your hands to form a cookie-like shape and arrange small cookies on the baking sheet you previously lined with parchment paper.
4. Bake for 15 minutes at the set temperature. Allow it to cool down before serving.

Skillet Brownies
Serves 4

Ingredients

1 egg

1/3 cup cocoa powder

1/3 cup Swerve or sweetener of your choice

7 tablespoons butter

1 tablespoon peanut butter

¼ cup almond flour

¼ cup walnuts

½ teaspoon baking powder

½ teaspoon vanilla extract

Salt to taste

Directions

1. Turn your oven to 350F to preheat it. Use a small saucepan to melt 6 tablespoons of butter over low-medium heat. Add Swerve or sweetener of your choice and let it dissolve in the butter.
2. Use a mixing bowl and combine butter-sweetener mixture with cocoa powder, vanilla extract, and salt to taste. Next, add the egg and use an electric hand mixer to mix everything well.
3. Add baking powder and almond flour and allow it to sit for 5 minutes for the dough to rise a bit.
4. Transfer the batter to the skillet and put it in the oven. Bake for 30 minutes at the set temperature.
5. In the meantime, combine peanut butter with the remaining tablespoon of butter to make a topping. Once the brownie is baked, top with the butter mix and serve.

Keto Coco Bark
Serves 6

Ingredients

½ cup coconut butter

½ cup coconut flakes

½ cup almonds

1 cup dark chocolate

10 drops liquid stevia

½ teaspoon almond extract

Salt to taste

Directions

1. Turn your oven to 350F to preheat it. Use parchment paper to line the baking sheet. Place the coconut flakes and almonds on the sheet and toast them for 7 minutes at the set temperature. Transfer it to a bowl.
2. Use a boiler to melt the chocolate and the coconut butter. Add liquid stevia and almond extract and combine everything well.
3. Use parchment paper to line the baking sheet again. Pour the melted chocolate on the sheet and use a spoon to spread it out evenly. Add coconut flakes and almonds on top and press them into the chocolate gently with your hands. Add salt to taste.
4. Put it in the fridge for at least 60 minutes to cool down before serving.

Choco Low-Carb Bar
Serves 6

Ingredients

1 egg

1 cup macadamias

1 cup sunflower seeds

1 cup almonds

1 cup coconut flakes

¼ cup peanut butter

¼ cup coconut butter

2 tablespoons vanilla extract

½ cup dark chocolate chips

1 teaspoon pumpkin pie spice

Directions

1. Turn your oven to 350F to preheat it. Use a blender or a food processor and add macadamias, almonds, sunflower seeds, coconut flakes, egg, coconut butter, peanut butter, dark chocolate chips, vanilla extract, and pumpkin pie spice. Process everything for about 3-4 seconds until you just incorporate the ingredients.
2. Transfer the mixture into a shallow heatproof dish. Spread it evenly and bake for 15 minutes at the set temperature. Allow it to cool down before serving.

Cheese Crackers
Serves 20

Ingredients

1 egg

2 cups Parmesan cheese

2 ounces cream cheese

1 cup almond flour

1 teaspoon rosemary

½ teaspoon salt

Directions

1. Use a heatproof bowl and add Parmesan cheese, cream cheese, and almond flour to it. Place it in the microwave and cook for 60 seconds or until you melt the cheese. Stir everything to make sure you combine the flour with the cheeses. Allow it to cool down.
2. Once it is cool enough, add egg, rosemary, and salt. Combine everything together well.
3. Use parchment paper to line a baking sheet. Wash your hands and use them to form a small ball from the batter and place it on the sheet. Continue until there is no more batter remaining.
4. Use a spatula or your palm to thin the balls and make a cookie-like form from them. Bake for 5 minutes at 450F before flipping them and cooking for additional 5 minutes. Allow them to cool down before serving.

Ketogenic Nachos
Serves 6

Ingredients

1 egg

2 tablespoon cream cheese

¾ cup almond flour

1 ¾ cups Mozzarella cheese, grated

1 teaspoon coriander powder

1 teaspoon cumin powder

½ teaspoon chili powder

Salt to taste

Sauce:

1 lb. minced beef

1 red onion

14 ounces can tomatoes

1 tablespoon tomato paste

¼ teaspoon chili powder

Directions

1. Let's make the sauce first. Use a small sauce pan and add some olive oil to it. Heat it to medium temperature and add the sliced red onion. Fry until it gets translucent and then add minced beef. Cook for about 5 minutes.
2. Add chili powder, tomato paste, and sliced canned tomatoes. Allow it to simmer for about 15 minutes over low heat. You want to get a smooth consistency.
3. In the meantime, use a heatproof bowl and add almond flour and Mozzarella cheese to it. Once you mix them, add the cream cheese. Place everything in the microwave for 60 seconds or more until you melt the cheeses.
4. Add egg, salt, coriander powder, chili powder, and cumin powder and mix everything together well.
5. Use parchment paper to line a baking sheet. Add the dough to the sheet and put another piece of parchment paper over it. Roll the dough into an even rectangle. Take out the top piece of the parchment paper.
6. Bake the batter for 15 minutes at 425F. Flip and cook for about 10 minutes on the other side (you want it to be brown on top).
7. Cut into triangle shapes that remind you of nachos. Bake for about 4 more minutes.
8. Arrange the nachos on a serving plate. Use a spoon to pour the meat sauce over them. Optionally, you can add more grated cheese on top.

Zucchini Mini Pizza
Serves 6

Ingredients

1 egg

1 cup Mozzarella cheese, shredded

½ cup Provolone cheese, grated

2 cups zucchini, shredded

¼ cup pepperoni slices

½ teaspoon oregano

½ teaspoon basil

Salt and pepper to taste

Directions

1. Turn your oven to 400F to preheat it. Use cooking spray to grease mini muffin pan.
2. Squeeze the liquid from the zucchini and place it in a bowl. Add egg, basil, oregano, Provolone cheese, and salt and pepper to taste to it. Combine all the ingredients well.
3. Transfer the mixture into the muffin molds, making sure to distribute it evenly across the tins. Use Mozzarella cheese to sprinkle over the zucchini mixture and then place pepperoni slices over it.
4. Bake for 15 minutes at the set temperature. Allow them to cool down before serving.

Get FREE Access To

"Pros & Cons of The Ketogenic Diet"

Go to: http://bit.ly/2rrnEM1

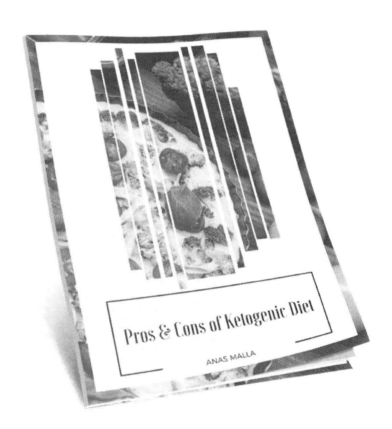

Conclusion

Thank you again for purchasing this book!

I hope this book was able to help you in preparing great recipes for your ketogenic diet plan. As you could see, most of the recipes are extremely easy to prepare, and they do not require advanced cooking knowledge. I tried to select a wide variety of recipes so that you can choose the ones that perfectly fit your taste.

The next step is to try out the various recipes. I'm sure you will be able delighted with a lot of them.

Finally, if you enjoyed this book, then I'd like to ask you for a favor, would you be kind enough to leave a review for this book on Amazon? It'd be greatly appreciated.

Visit the link below to leave a review:
https://www.amazon.com/review/create-review

For more information, please check out my blog at: Mastering-life.com

Thank you and good luck!

Preview of "Ketogenic Bread Cookbook"

Introduction

We are a society that is so used to eating wheat products; from bread to waffles and muffins such that when we learn that we need to give up some of these foods if you want to adopt the ketogenic diet, many simply think that the diet is not for them. The amazing thing is that just because you cannot have bread made from wheat and other grains, does not mean that you cannot have some bread. You can still make bread, muffins, waffles and breadsticks using other flours like almond flour, coconut flour and flax meal among others.

Are you looking to adopt the ketogenic diet and still want to enjoy some bread, muffins, or waffles? Are you tired of the usual breads and muffins made from wheat and want to enjoy other types of bread made using different kinds of flours? If this is what you are looking for; then look no further because in this book, you will learn some amazing bread, muffin, waffle, and breadstick recipes that you can prepare. Thanks to this book, you can still enjoy some bread and waffles even when on a ketogenic diet.

Thanks again for downloading this book, I hope you enjoy it!

Preparing ketogenic waffles, muffins, breads, breadsticks etc. revolves around replacing the flour used. Since on a ketogenic diet, you cannot eat grains, wheat is out of the question. However, you can replace wheat with almond flour, coconut flour, flaxseed among other flours. In addition, you cannot use sugar; thus, you will be replacing sugar with sweeteners like Erythritol, Stevia, Monk fruit powder etc. Your goal is to ensure that your daily net carbohydrate intake is around 40G or even less.

Let us now look at some tasty ketogenic recipes:

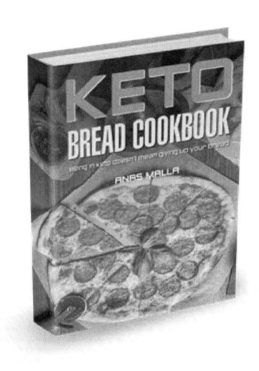

Bread Recipes
Cinnamon Bread

Serving Size: 10 slices

Ingredients

3 pastured eggs

1 teaspoon vinegar

3 tablespoons salted butter

2 tablespoons water

1/2 cup coconut flour

1/2 teaspoon baking soda

1 teaspoon cinnamon

1/2 teaspoon baking powder

1/3 cup pure sour cream or Greek Yogurt

1/8 teaspoon stevia or sweetener of choice

Directions

Preheat the oven to 350 degrees F.

Oil the loaf pan then line the bottom with parchment paper.

Mix the dry ingredients using a whisk until well blended. Add the rest of the ingredients to the dry mixture and mix well. Taste for sweetness and if needed, adjust. Let the mixture stand for 3 minutes then mix again.

Spread the batter onto the prepared loaf pan and bake for around 25-30 minutes until when you insert a toothpick at the centre it comes out clean.

Cool the loaf on a wire rack then store in the refrigerator.

Cinnamon Bread						
Ingredients	Calories	Carbs	Fat	Protein	Sodium	Sugar
Servings Per Recipe: 10 Servings						
3 pastured eggs	210	0	15	18	210	0
1 teaspoon vinegar	2	0	0	0	0	0
3 tablespoons salted butter	306	0	45	0	5	0
1/2 cup coconut flour	240	32	8	8	120	4
1/2 teaspoon baking soda	0	0	0	0	640	0
1 teaspoon cinnamon	6	2	0	0	0	0
1/2 teaspoon baking powder	0	0	0	0	200	0
1/3 cup pure sour cream	162	3	16	2	40	0
1/8 teaspoon stevia	0	0	0	0	0	0
Total:	926	37	84	28	1215	4
Per Serving:	93	4	8	3	122	0

Go to this link to check out the rest of the "**Ketogenic Bread Cookbook**":

http://amzn.to/2m8hixm

Check Out My Other Books

Below you'll find some of my other popular books that are popular on Amazon and Kindle as well. Simply click on the links below to check them out.

Alternatively, you can visit my "Author Page" on Amazon to see other work done by me:

Anas Malla: http://amzn.to/2nzCevB

- **Alkaline Diet V.1**
  http://amzn.to/2shityl
- **Ketogenic Diet**
  http://amzn.to/2ps3ePm
- **Ketogenic Bread Cookbook V.1**
  http://amzn.to/2m8hixm
- **Ketogenic Bread Cookbook V.2**
  http://amzn.to/2r3qsPJ
- **Ketogenic Bread Cookbook V.3**
  http://amzn.to/2r3Af8j
- **Instant Pot Ketogenic Cookbook V.1**
  http://amzn.to/2o4oCfP
- **Instant Pot Ketogenic Cookbook V.2**
  http://amzn.to/2o4oCfP
- **Ketogenic Fat Bombs V.1**
  http://amzn.to/2qDgS4U
- **Minimalist Living**
  http://amzn.to/2phTu8M
- **Conversation Tactics**
  http://amzn.to/2oj23Qg

If the links do not work, for whatever reason, you can simply search for these titles on the Amazon website to find them.

Made in the USA
Lexington, KY
11 August 2017